The Magic of Green Tea

Green Tea for Health

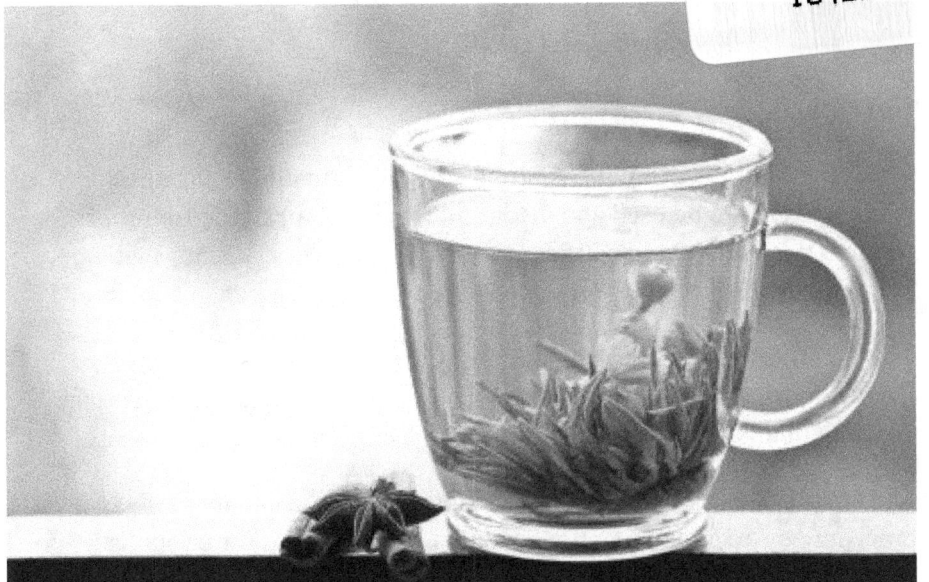

Dueep Jyot Singh

Healthy Living Series

Mendon Cottage Books

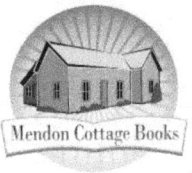

JD-Biz Publishing

Download Free Books!

http://MendonCottageBooks.com

Disclaimer

The information is this book is provided for informational purposes only. It is not intended to be used and medical advice or a substitute for proper medical treatment by a qualified health care provider. The information is believed to be accurate as presented based on research by the author.

The contents have not been evaluated by the U.S. Food and Drug Administration or any other Government or Health Organization and the contents in this book are not to be used to treat cure or prevent disease.

The author or publisher is not responsible for the use or safety of any diet, procedure or treatment mentioned in this book. The author or publisher is not responsible for errors or omissions that may exist.

Warning

The Book is for informational purposes only and before taking on any diet, treatment or medical procedure, it is recommended to consult with your primary health care provider.

Our books are available at

1. Amazon.com

2. Barnes and Noble

3. Itunes

4. Kobo

5. Smashwords

6. Google Play Books

Table of Contents

Introduction

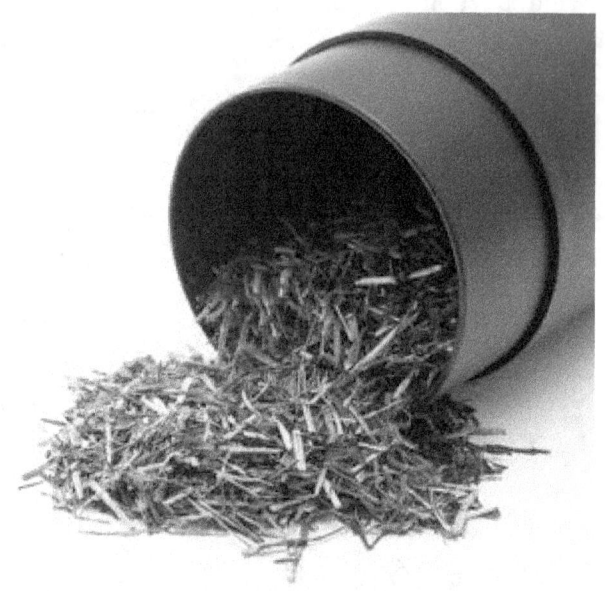

Since ancient times, man has been looking for healthy drinks, which could promote good health, longevity, and vitality. Green tea comes in this category.

A majority of us cannot do without the cup that cheers, early in the morning. Sometimes we may even find ourselves addicted to our cup of hearty java, first thing in the morning before we can wake up completely.

But since ancient times, green tea has been such a major part of the lives of people who are very careful about their health, that it is no wonder that it is one of the most popular of natural healthy drinks going in the world today.

The ancient Chinese preferred going without food rather than forfeit their cup of refreshing "Cha". That is because tea was such a major part of Chinese culture in ancient times, that tea drinking ceremonies which were then adapted by Japan, were a major part of the social fabric. Even today, there are exotic teas which are going for thousands of dollars on the auction table, because they are considered to be such rare, distinguished and exotic beverages.

Of the three major beverages of the world, tea is definitely the most popular. "Cha" is a word which is recognized all over the world, especially when one demands something refreshing to drink after a hard days' work at the office or sitting doing that hard days' work in the office.

History of Tea

Historically, tea has been assimilated in the social fabric for millenniums. Serendipity has a great hand in the knowledge of tea, like that of coffee. Coffee was supposedly found by a shepherd who had seen his goats eating some berries off a bush and then acting in a very enthusiastic and frisky manner.

In the same way tea was supposedly discovered by a Chinese Emperor more than 3000 years ago. He was sitting in his garden and a few leaves of a fragrant camellia bush accidentally fell into a cauldron of boiling water in the vicinity. The resulting fragrance tempted the Emperor to sip this refreshing brew. And soon everybody in China was steeping the leaves of the Camellia in hot water and drinking the resulting infusion down.

It was only later that the proper preparation of tea, in the form of drying the leaves, fermentation, oxidization and other tea preparation methods before it was packaged and sold to the consumers, became known globally down the ages.

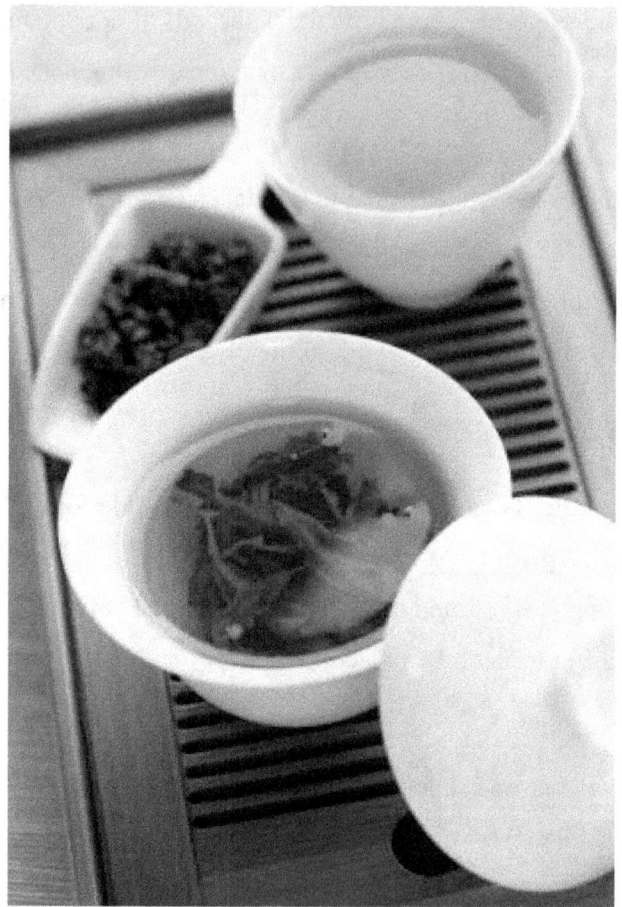

The Camellia sinensis plant is normally used for the preparation of green tea. The tea available in the market is normally found in 3 forms – black tea, green tea and oolong tea. All these teas are made through different phases of drying and intensity of the fermentation process.

About 3 billion kgs of tea are consumed all over the world annually, of which the major tea drinkers are the Chinese, Japanese, Indians, which come up to 43% of the world population of tea drinkers.

In ancient Eastern medicine, tea has been used as a relaxant, and healing drink. According to the Chinese, drinking lots of tea meant that you would not suffer from stomach problems, headaches, nervous tension, and any other disease, of which you could think. For the last 4000 years, tea has been an important ingredient used to cure people in alternative medicines in the East.

This is normally given to the patient in either an infusion form where it is allowed to steep in water for a long time, or in decoction forms, when herbs are added to the mixture, allowed to steep and then given to the patient.

How to recognize Green Tea

Green tea is easily recognizable because of its greenish color, even though it is powdered dried tea leaves, packed for you. Proper tea preparation is done through fermenting the leaves and allowing them either to dry in the sun or go through an oxidation process. However, green tea is not fermented before being packaged and marketed. That is why all the powerful natural antioxidants which were lost to other teas during the fermentation process still remain present in natural green tea.

This also means that it is going to have a more delicate taste than fermented and oxidized black tea. Nevertheless, it is steamed and rolled before it is dried and packaged. The original color of the tea leaves without fermentation is going to be kept depending on the variety of the green tea plant and species.

How to Prepare Green Tea

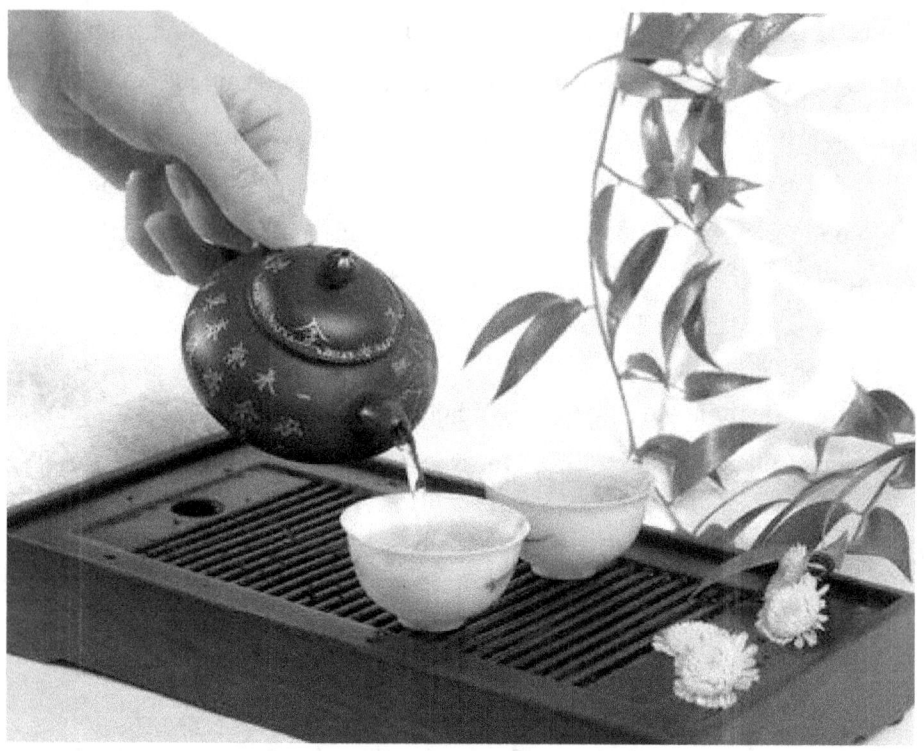

To prepare green tea all you need to do is take 1 teaspoon of green tea leaves for one cup of water which is just below boiling temperature.

Let it steep for 10 minutes and then strain. You may add lemon or honey according to your taste. Do not add milk. The tea is to be sipped slowly and not gulped down.

Today. Green tea is commercially available all over the world and is a very popular gift. The only side effect of green tea is that like coffee, it is going to induce insomnia. Hence, it is advisable to take the evening cup of tea at least 3 or 4 hours before your bedtime. That means you are giving yourself plenty of opportunity to feel totally tired out by the time you are ready to go to sleep.

Ideally one should have 10 cups of green tea a day in order to get all its benefits. Green tea capsules are available in the market, but like I said before they are pretty expensive and are definitely not going to give you the same benefit which is given to you by the original thing.

Green tea extracts are now getting to be very popular with weight loss products manufacturers. They have also found a place in cholesterol-lowering drugs. You can also find them in dietary supplements, breakfast foods, beauty products and beverages available all over the world. Lipton, a world-famous producer of black and green tea has begun packaging bottles of green tea as a cool refreshing drink and going against soft drink giants like Coca-Cola and Pepsi in the process.

Health Benefits of Green Tea

For millenniums people have been using green tea as one of the best detoxifying agents present in the world today. Many Orientals and easterners on the average drink one – 2 cups per day as a cleanser for the body. According to them, this is the best detoxifying agent available to you from the bounty of nature. Though for longer lasting effects, you will need to drink anywhere between 6 to 8 cups of tea every day.

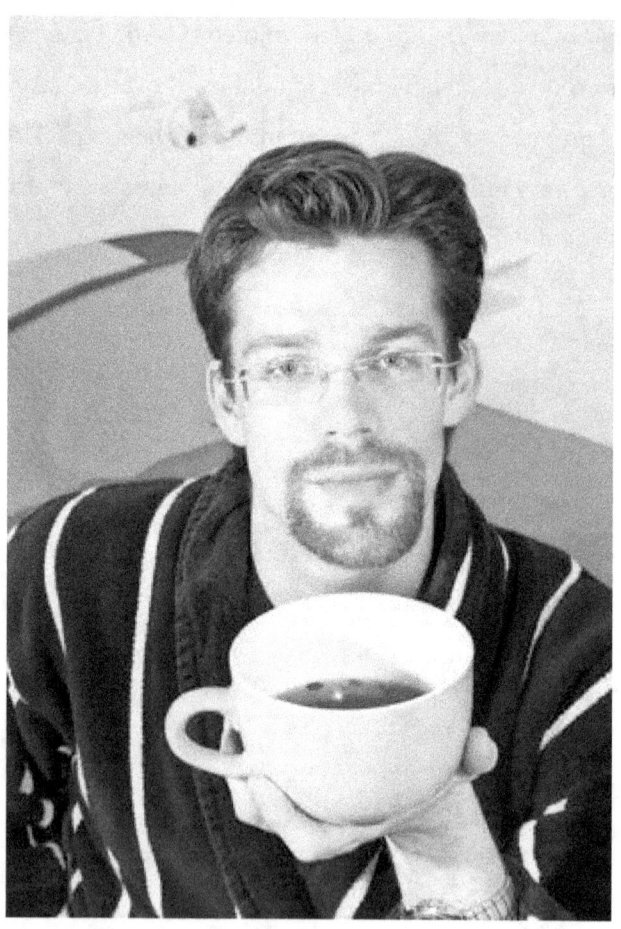

The only positive thing I can say about this suggestion of an elevated tea intake is that you are never going to suffer from dehydration and also, you are not going to suffer from kidney problems, because green tea is an excellent diuretic!

One of the reasons why green tea is supposed to be so I healthy is because they have catechins which have excellent disease fighting and health restoring properties.

Being powerful antioxidants, these catechins have been shown in recent studies to be able to fight viruses as well as bacteria. But we do not need research to tell us something our ancestors new thousands of years ago. Green tea has been used to ward off cough and cold and also infections for centuries, in the shape of a brew or decoction.

Also, green tea was considered by the ancients as the best way in which they could slow the aging process. It also had a beneficial effect on general health. In fact, if you are suffering from cough and cold during the winter, just start drinking lots of green tea. You will not have to bother much about the vitamin C and vitamin E intake then.

Vitamin E is one of the necessary ingredients needed by your body to keep your hair and skin healthy and glowing. So with that green tea intake, you are going to have a signal improvement in the texture and quality of your skin and hair.

This is the reason why I have given some beauty recipes below, which are going to improve the quality of your skin as well as your hair. You can bless the vitamin E for that.

Best Detoxifying Agent

Apart from water being one of the best ingredients in nature to help detoxify your body, the inclusion of green tea leaves is an added benefit. This tea when taken in great quantities throughout the day is capable of fighting all the free radicals present in your body. These free radicals cause a number of diseases. These diseases are thus prevented by the antioxidants present in green tea.

That is why more and more research is being done on how green tea is capable of promoting good health as it has done in centuries.

We being a cynical breed are definitely not going to listen to what are ancients told us. We would rather have a well-qualified scientist with a number of alphabets behind his name tell us something which has already been known, in order that it become acceptable to us. Also billions of dollars are being wasted on research on a thing which has already been known. But then, the idea of a fool and his money and somebody else is going to party...

Cardiovascular Diseases

Green tea has a number of antioxidants. These are capable of preventing high blood pressure, cholesterol, and even blood clots. That is how they protect the body against cardiovascular diseases. The catechins slow down the

Drinking lots of green tea means that you are going to improve cholesterol ratio for low-density lipoprotein cholesterol and high density lipoprotein cholesterol. Also, all the fibrinogen content as well as the triglycerides content, which are conducive in causing possible heart ailments are going to be lowered in your body, after you drink lots of green tea. All of these are blood indicators of any possible heart disease in human beings and animals. Thus, it is going to help in reducing the cholesterol level.

I remember an ex-boss of mine, who had a terrible temper. In fact, half of the fun of working there was to take bets when he would go off in an apoplexy or a stroke, because he would get into tempers at the slightest provocation, and go all red in his face like a turkey cock.

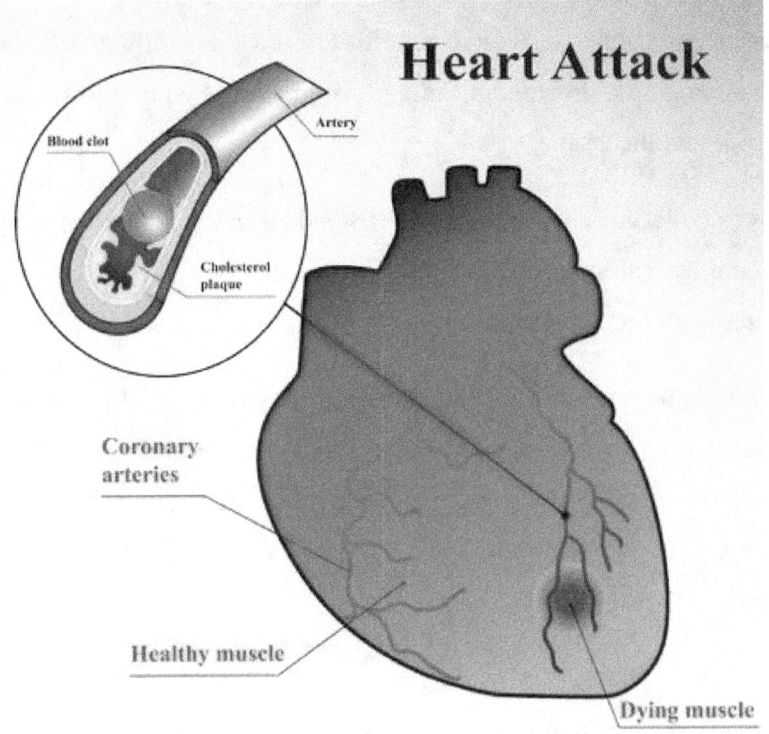

If you think that you are vulnerable to heart disease, add green tea to your diet immediately.

One fine day, his lady wife decided that she had got a bit tired of his uncontrollable bad temper, which was not doing her blood pressure or his blood pressure any good. So she switched him onto green tea. Though it did not have any visible effect on his bad temper, – because he was one of those spoilt kids who never grew up and thought shouting and bullying was the only way in which he could get his orders obeyed – there was a significant lowering of his blood pressure levels.

Even though I am not a tea drinker, nor a coffee drinker, this idea that green tea could be used as an antioxidant, as well as a stress buster took great precedence in the health-related priorities of the whole office. So I had to watch them guzzle down huge amounts of green tea, while I just inhaled the fragrance and the aroma.

All those colleagues are in their late 40s and 50s now. And all of them are quite healthy with no problems of heart or diabetes and all of them keep drinking lots of green tea.

Let me tell you one amusing side benefit of drinking lots of green tea. It is capable of keeping your teeth healthy! That is because it has plenty of fluoride in it. It kills all the bacteria that cause dental plaque. It also checks the dental decay by inhibiting the growth of oral bacteria and so it fights cavities.

That is why, when we were young and suffered from the rare case of toothache, we were immediately told to gargle and rinse our mouths with lots of green tea solution. In fact I have seen a number of people drinking green tea first thing in the morning, and then swishing the liquid around in their mouths and spitting it out. According to them, this cleans their teeth beforehand before they go to brush and floss their teeth.

Also, people suffering from halitosis should rinse their mouths out with green tea solutions as often as possible. This is going to keep the breath fresh and sweet.

You can also use it as a toothpaste substitute by 5 tablespoons full of green tea and steeping them in quarter cup of boiling hot water for about half an hour. Then put all the leaves in your compost heap and use the liquid to make a toothpaste. This is done by adding 1 teaspoon each of finely powdered salt and soda bicarbonate/baking soda. This is your toothpaste which you are going to use to brush your teeth, and get rid of halitosis as well as plaque.

Stress Buster

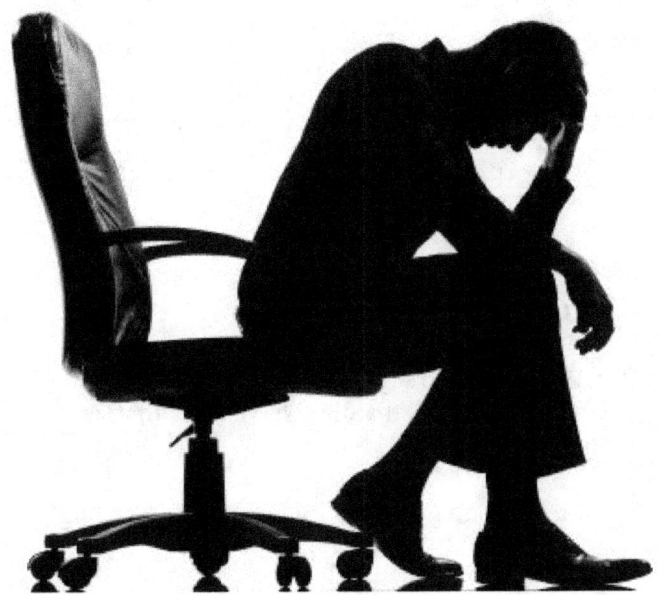

Catechin present in green tea is capable of removing lethargy and sleepiness. It also works as a stress buster. If you are in need of an extra boost, just drink green tea, instead of coffee with its addictive caffeine content. Green tea is a better stimulant for short time energy. The drink has got a diuretic effect.

A green tea solution is also a good antiseptic, because all you have to do is wipe an affected wound, scratch, or skin ailment with a green tea solution. This cures it. When a friend of mine told me that her grandmother had learned this from her grandmother, I naturally scoffed and told her that this was the easiest way in which people could keep clean and prevent bacterial infections caused by poor hygiene and dirty conditions.

That is the reason why so many skin diseases, wounds, scratches, rashes, etc. have been healed with the cleansing solutions made up of water and herbs and also leaves like neem, marigold flowers and so on and so forth.

The microbes present in the body are capable of being destroyed by green tea, because of its very powerful antibiotic, antiviral and antibacterial properties.

Weight Loss through Green Tea

It is a wonder why people have not found out that green tea is capable of helping you lose weight. If you say, that they have done that, and they have not found it effective, it is possible that they are not following strict weight loss rules and are just relying on green tea to help them lose weight!

These people are quite capable of eating lots of fatty food, carbohydrates, and other food items contributing to plenty of fat and cellulite, and washing it all down with lots of green tea. Green tea does not have any calories at all, so apart from fresh fruit juice, you can use green tea as a weight loss drink.

It is supposed that green tea enhances the metabolic rate and prevents the digestion of carbohydrates. This is the reason why, any Japanese meal, which is rich in carbohydrates is going to be accompanied with lots of green tea before, during and after the meal. This has been done for centuries, and is still followed today.

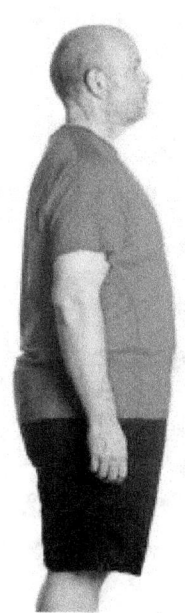 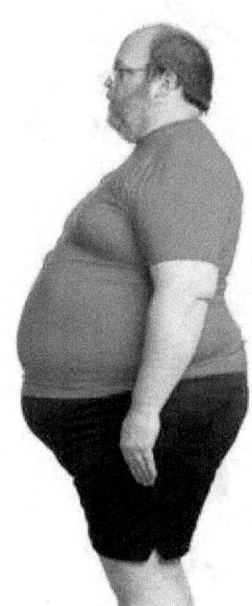

So the next time you eat something rich in carbohydrates, you may want to drink lots of green tea as a refreshing accompaniment.

Cancer Fighting Properties

According to researchers, green tea is capable of preventing a number of cancers, including stomach cancer. Cancerous cells were experimented on with extracts of green tea and their growth stopped or was inhibited. This experiment was done in 2004. According to these findings and facts, the researchers decided that green tea had some powerful ingredient which would target the growth of cancerous cells, and prevent them from growing or proliferating any further.

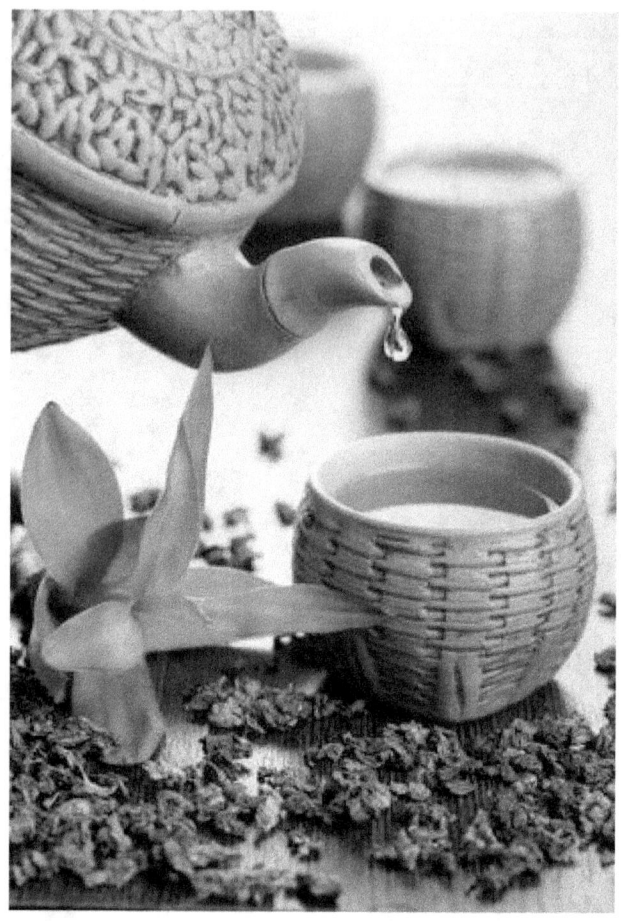

These researchers also requested researchers in Japan to collaborate with them, on this particular study, researching the reasons why the incidence of cancer is so low in Japan. This was because of the excessive green tea consumption. It has now been proven through clinical and animal studies that EGC was responsible for playing an important role in the prevention of any types of cancer. These included breast cancer, skin cancer, lung cancer, stomach cancer, prostate cancer, ovary and colon cancer.

Antiaging Properties

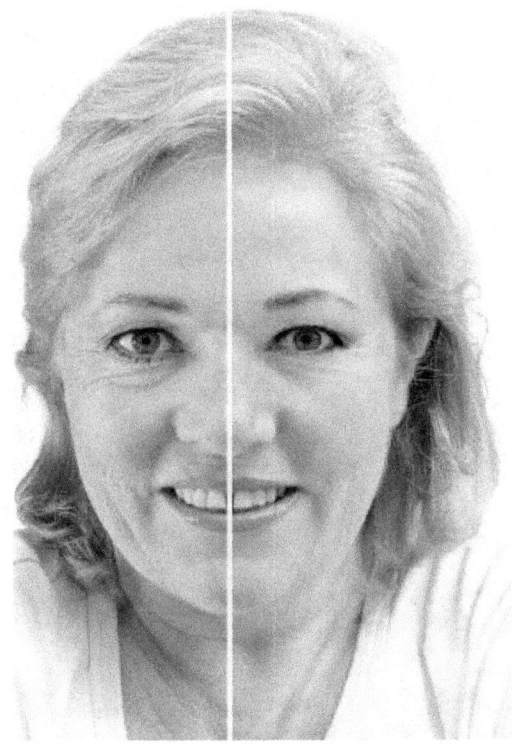

Nowadays, many antiaging remedies are putting in green tea extract and selling them to the public. Seriously, a green tea extract along with a large number of other ingredients and chemical fillers are definitely not going to be as beneficial to you, even if they come packaged in a very expensive and well advertised packet. Instead, make a cup of green tea from lots of fresh green tea leaves, and drink it down with lemon, milk and honey.

Green tea has the ability of feeling your body really quickly. That is because it boosts up your immunity system. It delays aging by the strong antioxidant action which prevents the accumulation of free radicals. These free radical are capable of damaging the DNA and thus causing aging.

So logic says that if you are worried about free radical build up in your body, drink lots of green tea.

Other Health Benefits

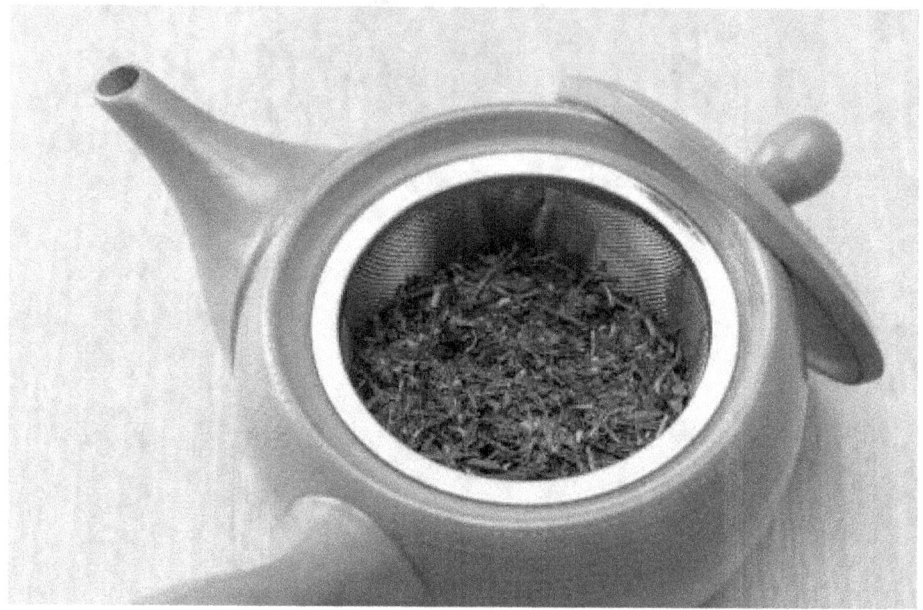

Since ancient times, people knew that green tea was responsible of preventing any infections in the joints. Also, inflamed joints could get relief with hot fomentation with green tea as well as drinking of it.

It is also believed to help boost immunity with its stimulating effect on the immune system. In ancient Chinese, Japanese and Korean cuisine, green tea played such an important role, that any meal served without green tea was considered to be incomplete.

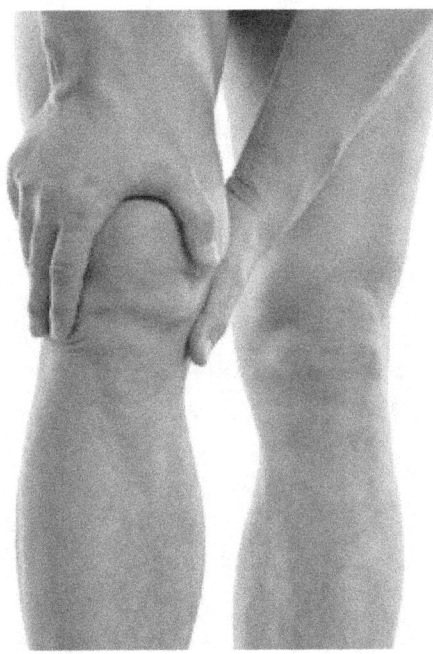

Green tea can greatly improve joint mobility.

That is because the wise men of yore knew that it would act as an herbalist for aiding in the circulation of blood. It also detoxified the body, and the blood and acted as an aid in curing liver ailments.

In fact I found green tea as a part of the diet in drug and alcohol rehabilitation and detoxification institutions. This green tea had fennel seeds added to it, and it was followed up with fresh orange juice. According to her doctor friend who was working there, the fennel as well as the orange juice managed to tackle the craving for alcohol, especially when the patient was going through withdrawal.

Green tea was useful for detoxifying the body, building up the immunity system, and getting the body back to normal without the poisonous toxins produced in the body through years of alcohol abuse.

Green Tea as a Beauty Aid

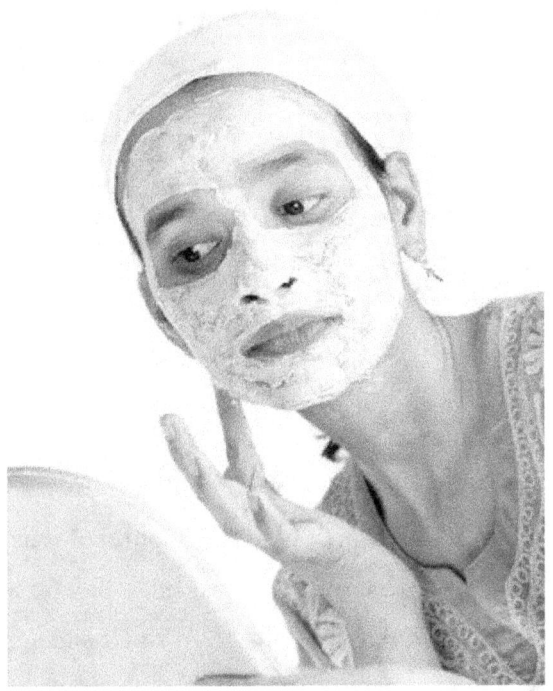

Many beauty product – manufacturing companies have now begun to include green tea extract in the recipe for beauty. Recent research suggests that green tea is capable of protecting your skin against the damage causing by ultraviolet rays and that is why they are being put in sunscreen creams. It is also used as a cooling agent, especially to fight the heat.

Apart from cooling your system down, it is going to give you a feeling of relaxation.

Green tea also has miraculous skin rejuvenating properties. The ancient Chinese and Japanese called green tea Green Jade.

Apply green tea solution on your eyes, when they are tired out. I normally use it as a fresher, with one teaspoonful of fresh mint leaves added to 6 teaspoons full of powdered green tea steeped for 20 minutes in a cup of boiling hot water. Allow it to cool down, put in your favorite spritzer – glass is perfect, plastic won't do, and spritz whenever you are feeling warm. You can also dip cards of cotton in the solution and put it over your tired eyes to relax and refresh them.

Here are some of my favorite recipes taken from ancient Chinese beauty books.[1]

Skin Rejuvenator

If you are looking for a good skin rejuvenator, blemish remover and anti-acne remedy, try this out. Mix 1 tablespoon full of freshly powdered green tea with one teaspoonful of honey, half a teaspoonful of lemon and the white of an egg. Spread it all over the affected areas and relax for as long as it takes until it dries up. Then remove with warm water and apply cold water to close the pores.

Do it every day, as long as you want, because after all, it is protecting your skin.

Mandy is close to 65 now, but she has a skin like a 25-year-old's. Surprising how more ancient Chinese recipes and Japanese beauty remedies have not managed to make their presence felt in the 21st-century beauty world today.

---

[1] I do not read Mandarin or Cantonese! I am indebted for these recipes to my friend Mandy Lu.

Also, according to her, this green tea has antiaging properties. Thanks to the pollution, exposure to harsh rays of the sun, and terrible lifestyle habits, all of us find ourselves aging rapidly, with sunspots, blemishes and wrinkles.

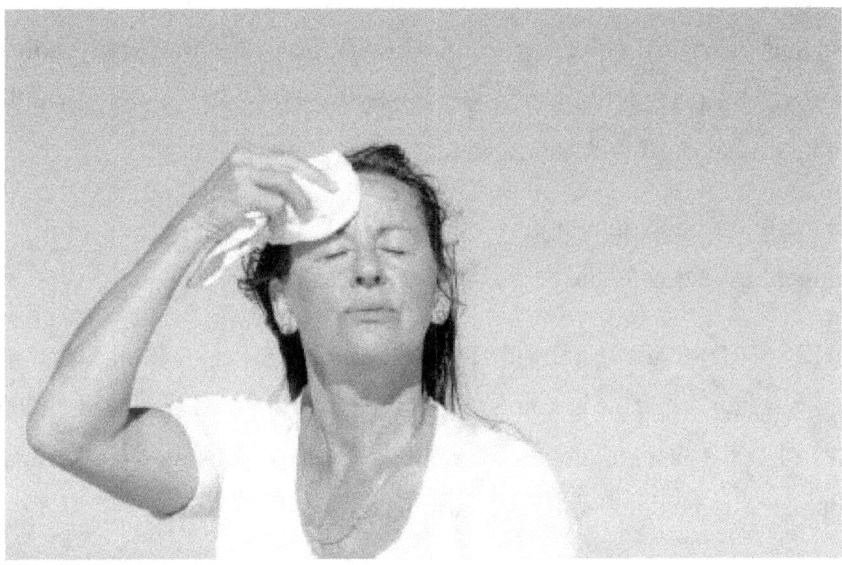

Apart from ECGC, green tea also has OPC – oligomeric pro – anthocyanidins, which are amazingly powerful and strong antioxidants. These are capable of preventing premature wrinkles, and aging signs. That is because they get rid of the toxins in your body, and prevent the free radicals from setting up shop and affecting your skin adversely.

Apart from this, the moment you find yourself washing your face after a green tea skin rejuvenator face mask, you are going to feel that it is softer and supple, smoother and younger looking.

That is because the elastin and the collagen tissue present in your skin are not broken down by enzymes, thanks to the effect of green tea. That is why your skin is going to feel smooth, and look really young and supple.

The antiaging facemask which I use on my face is made up of 1 tablespoon full of green tea powdered and mixed with 1 teaspoon of honey and 5 teaspoons of yogurt. The ancients used cream, but I do not want my skin to feel oily. This paste is allowed to dry on my face for 20 – 30 minutes and then it is washed off with warm water.

I normally use some lemon juice on top of this after washing as a mild astringent, and closing the pores.

You can also use this as a facial scrub by scrubbing it in a circular fashion when it is half dry. This is going to exfoliate the skin, and get rid of all that dust and grime accumulated throughout the day. Any rinsing which needs to be done has to be done with lukewarm water.

Getting Rid of Sunburn

I noticed that green tea, along with apple cider vinegar is extremely good for getting rid of any sort of sunburn, especially when you went out in the sun without proper covering. This is going to heal the skin, if you apply it directly to the area which has been affected.

Skin which has been sun damaged can be healed by some of the ingredients present in green tea. These include polyphenols, and tannic acid as well as theobromine. This is the reason why so many sunscreen manufacturers are adding green tea extracts to their products, as well as in their skin repair products. These polyphenols, etc. are capable of preventing any sort of inflammation in the damaged skin.

For this all you have to do is make up some green tea, allow it to infuse and freeze it. I normally freeze it in ice cube trays. Whenever I come home with my skin badly tanned and sunburned, I wrap the cubes in a cloth and apply slowly to the affected area. It cools down my skin even though I need to remove the sunburn with buttermilk later on.

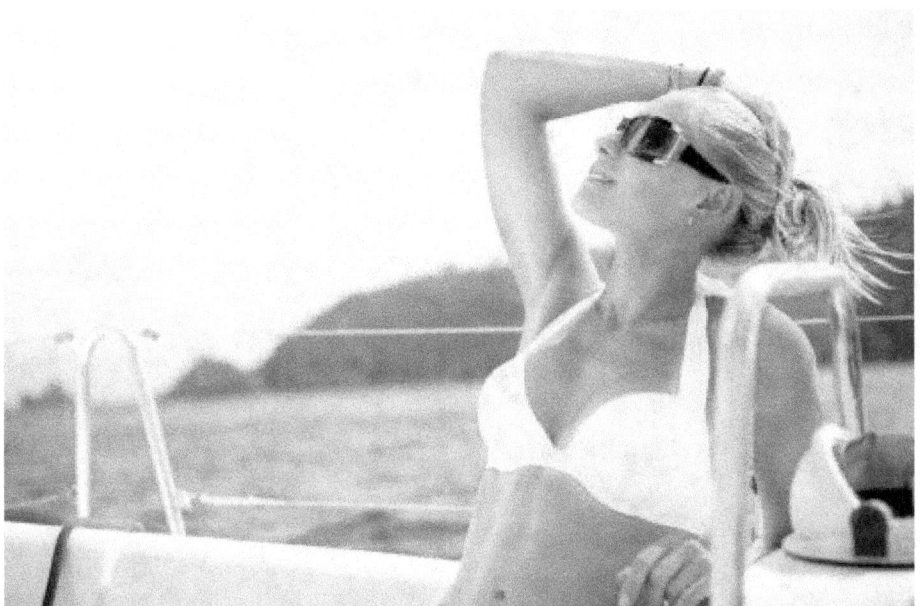

Green Tea for Your Hair

Green tea is an excellent natural product to keep your hair healthy, shiny, and prevent scalp diseases like dandruff, psoriasis, and even baldness. For this, you have to steep 5 spoonfuls of green tea in 4 cups of boiling hot water and allow to infuse for about half an hour. By that time you will have shampooed and condition your hair. I normally do not use any chemical conditioners on my hair and that is why I do not have gray hair even though I will never see 45 again.

My conditioning is normally done by massaging the scalp with warm coconut oil/olive oil/mustard oil – anything available – about 2 hours before I want to shampoo. I do not leave it overnight because I do not like my pillows stained with oil stains and I do not like covering my hair up in plastic shower caps while I am asleep.

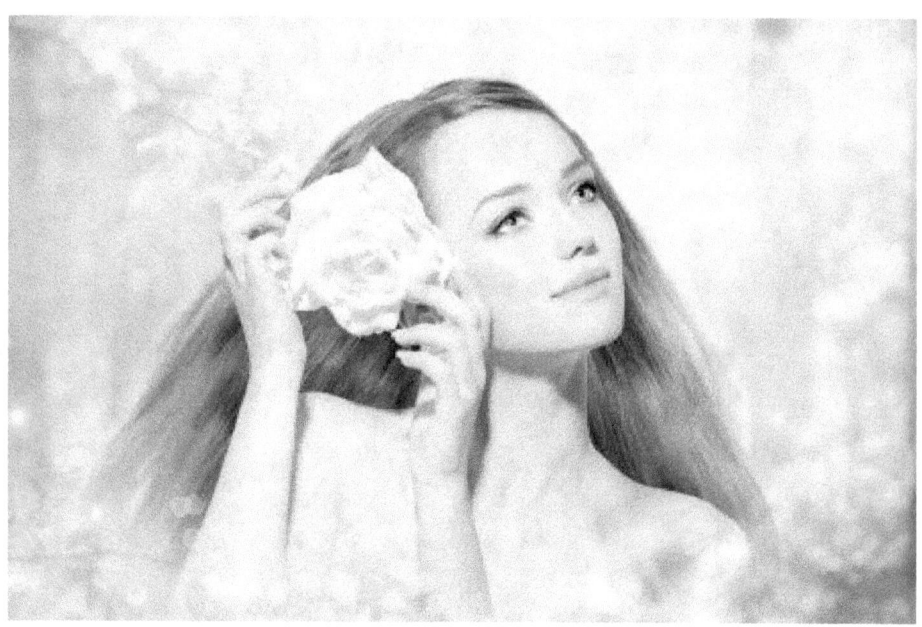

So after you have allowed your hair to be conditioned by the warm oil for about 2 hours or even more, – the longer it is, the silkier and more manageable your hair will be – shampoo it with a herbal powder – look for herbal powders with powdered gooseberry, soap nut and shikakai. You just need to apply one teaspoonful of this powder onto your hair, and wash off.

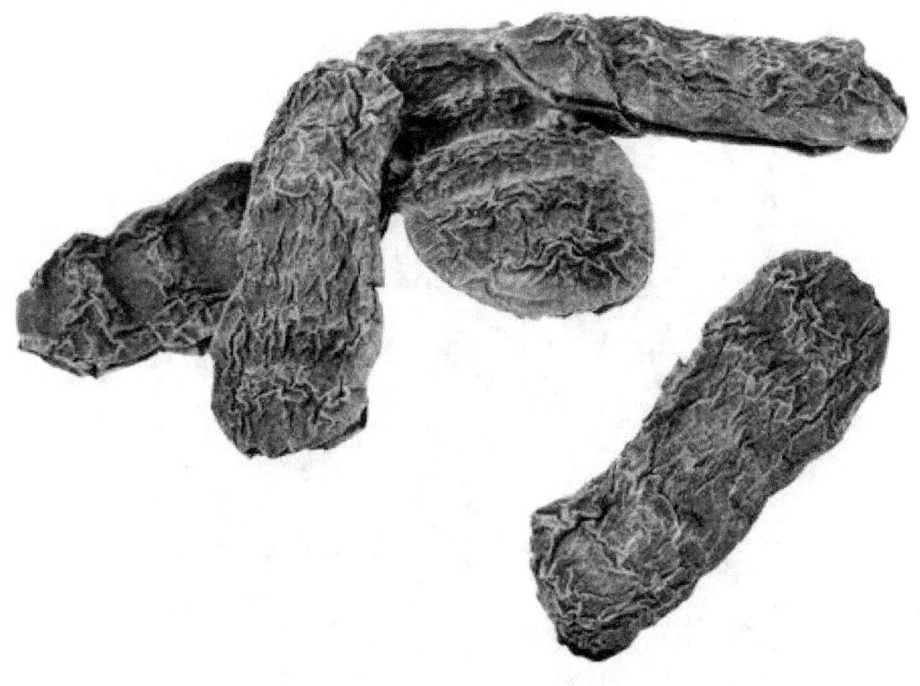

Shikakai- acacia concinna

Your hair are going to be washed clean due to the soap nut and stay there natural color due to the gooseberry and the shikakai. If you are a blonde, look for an herbal powder without shikakai and gooseberry, because it darkens the hair and prevents it from turning gray or white.

After that, here comes the conditioning with green tea. The last rinse is going to be done with the Tea solution. This is more powerful than beer or lemons/vinegar as a last rinse. And you are going to have silky, shiny, squeaky clean hair which are going to be your crowning glory.

Traditional Green Tea Home Cure Remedies

Basil leaf – green tea decoction

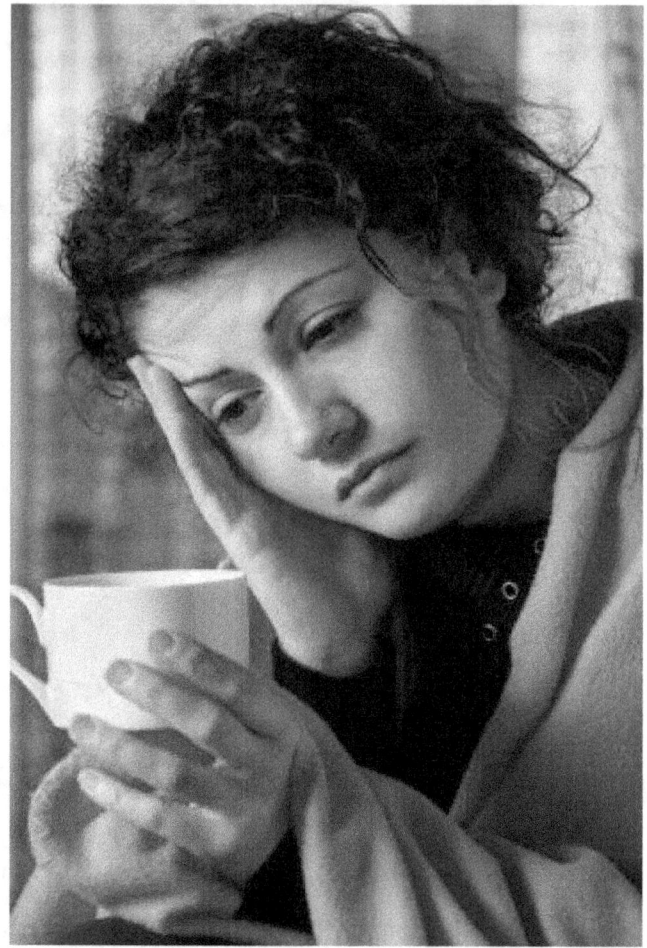

A recipe from The Indian Spice Kitchen, this is the surest cure for a persistent sore throat, cough and cold, and also makes for a refreshing herbal drink.

- 2 cardamoms

- 2 cloves

- 1 teaspoon cumin seeds

- 1 teaspoon fennel seeds

- 600 mL – 1 pint – water

- 2 teaspoons holy basil leaves, dried

- 1 teaspoon green leaf tea

- honey to taste.

Remove the cardamom seeds from their husks then crush them roughly with the cloves. In a heavy bottomed pan, dry roast the cloves, cardamoms, cumin and fennel seeds.

As soon as they start smoking at the water and the tea leaves. Allow them to boil before adding the basil leaves.

Shut of the heat and allow to steep for 2 or 3 minutes. Then switch on the heat again and bring to a boil for last-minute steeping.

Add honey for sweetener. Serve hot. This decoction is drank in the winter, in copious quantities, so that you get the full effect of the honey, spices, green tea and basil leaves. So, the moment you begin to start feeling cold, when you come home after battling from the harsh elements and feel a cold coming on, just make this, drink it down, wrap yourself up in a blanket and allow your body to cure itself. The incipient cold will have disappeared by morning.

Conclusion

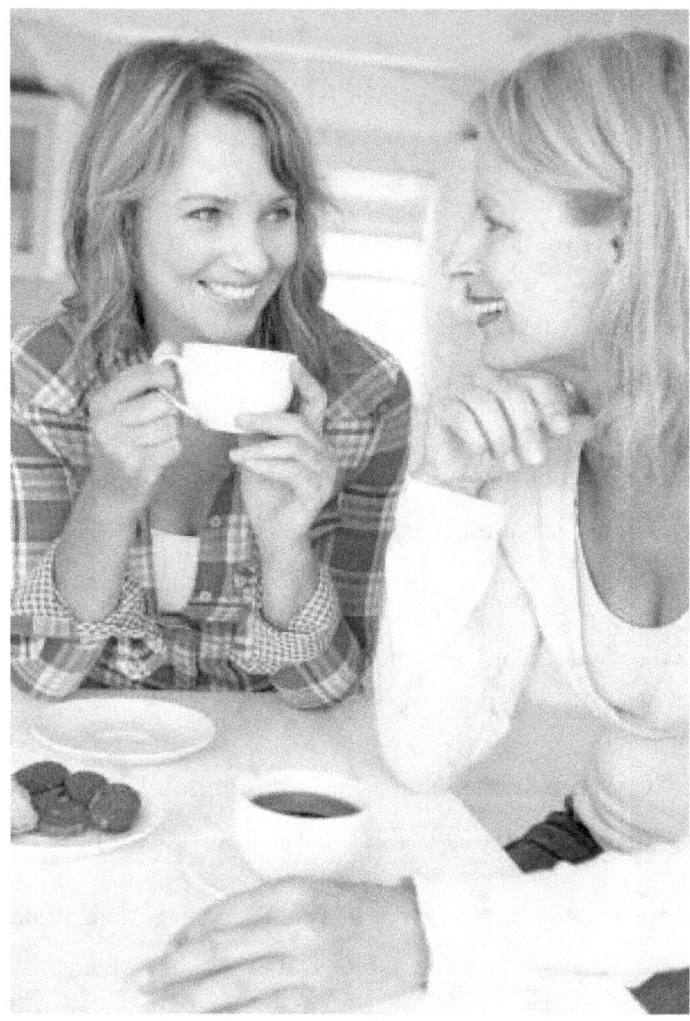

Few herbs go back in time, as much as tea does. Black tea, green tea and Oolong has been a daily necessity in many parts of the East and the Orient for millenniums, and the art of growing, processing, brewing and drinking the beverage evolved in China from where it spread to Japan and other parts of the world.

You are going to find a wide variety of brews adorning the supermarket shelves today. However, when you put green tea in your shopping basket, it is going to be a welcome addition to your stock of good health ingredients in your larder. Even though people in ancient times knew all about it, modern scientific research in both Asia and the West are still providing hard evidence of the health benefits associated with drinking green tea as often as possible.

So go ahead and enjoy this magical, healthy, refreshing and beneficial drink which has myriad therapeutic and medicinal properties, the knowledge of which has been passed down to us by the ancients down the ages.

Live Long and Prosper!

Author Bio

Dueep Jyot Singh is a Management and IT Professional who managed to gather Postgraduate qualifications in Management and English and Degrees in Science, French and Education while pursuing different enjoyable career options like being an hospital administrator, IT,SEO and HRD Database Manager/ trainer, movie , radio and TV scriptwriter, theatre artiste and public speaker, lecturer in French, Marketing and Advertising, ex-Editor of Hearts On Fire (now known as Solstice) Books Missouri USA, advice columnist and cartoonist, publisher and Aviation School trainer, ex-moderator on Medico.in, banker, student councilor ,travelogue writer … among other things!

One fine morning, she decided that she had enough of killing herself by Degrees and went back to her first love -- writing. It's more enjoyable! She already has 48 published academic and 14 fiction- in- different- genre books under her belt.

When she is not designing websites or making Graphic design illustrations for clients , she is browsing through old bookshops hunting for treasures, of which she has an enviable collection – including R.L. Stevenson, O.Henry, Dornford Yates, Maurice Walsh, De Maupassant, Victor Hugo, Sapper, C.N. Williamson, "Bartimeus" and the crown of her collection- Dickens "The Old Curiosity Shop," and "Martin Chuzzlewit" and so on… Just call her "Renaissance Woman") - collecting herbal remedies, acting like Universal Helping Hand/Agony Aunt, or escaping to her dear mountains for a bit of exploring, collecting herbs and plants and trekking.

Check out some of the other JD-Biz Publishing books

Gardening Series on Amazon

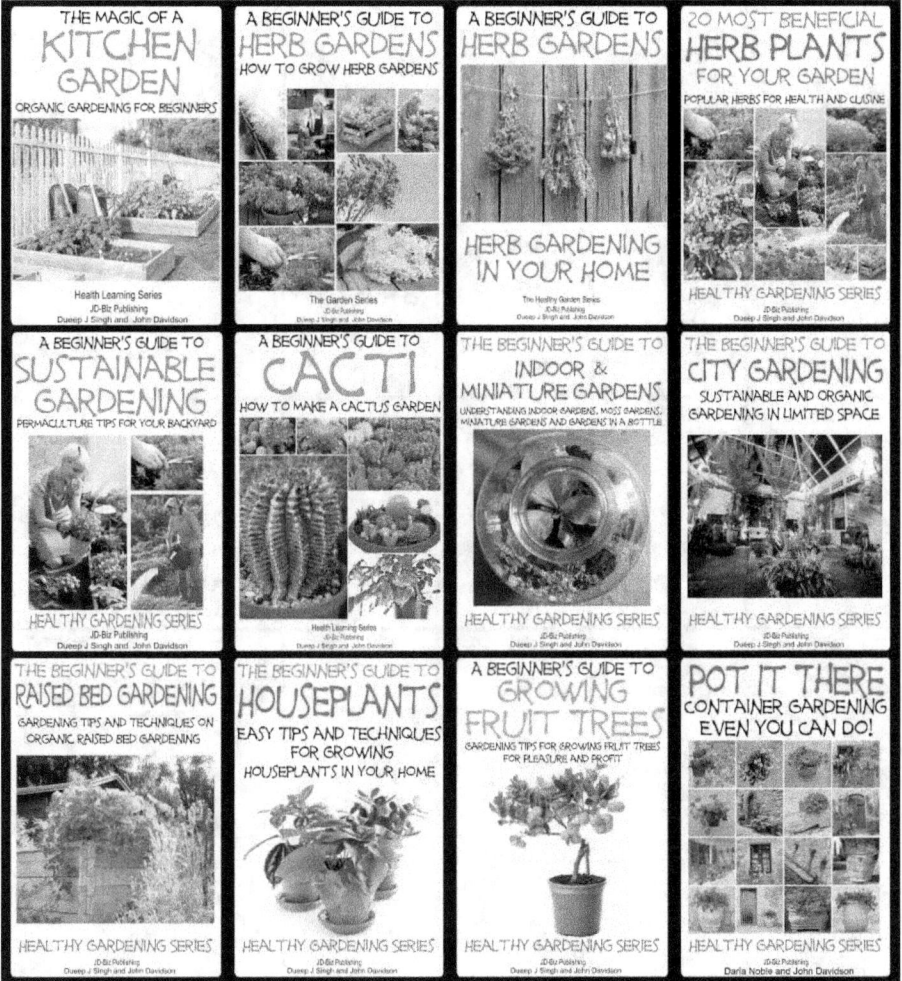

Download Free Books!

http://MendonCottageBooks.com

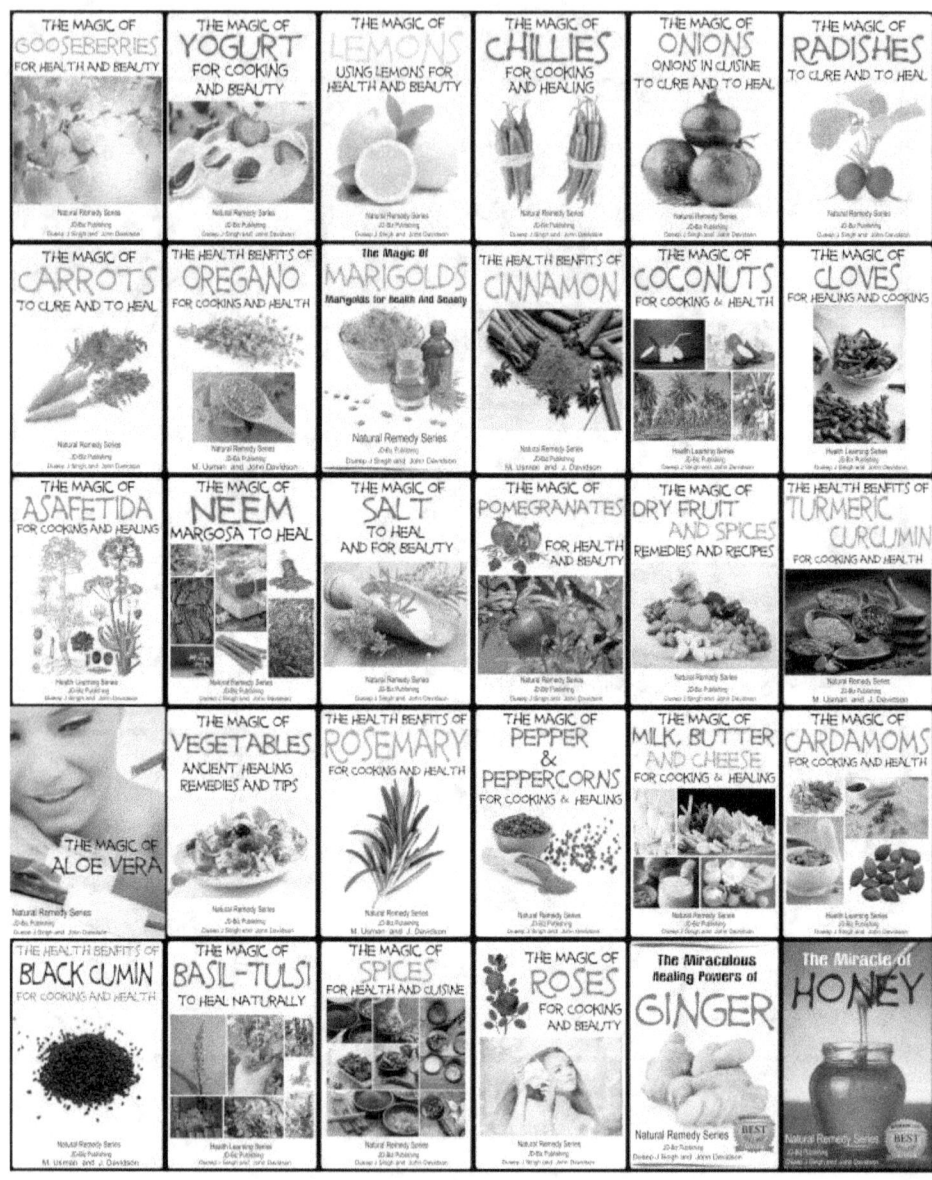

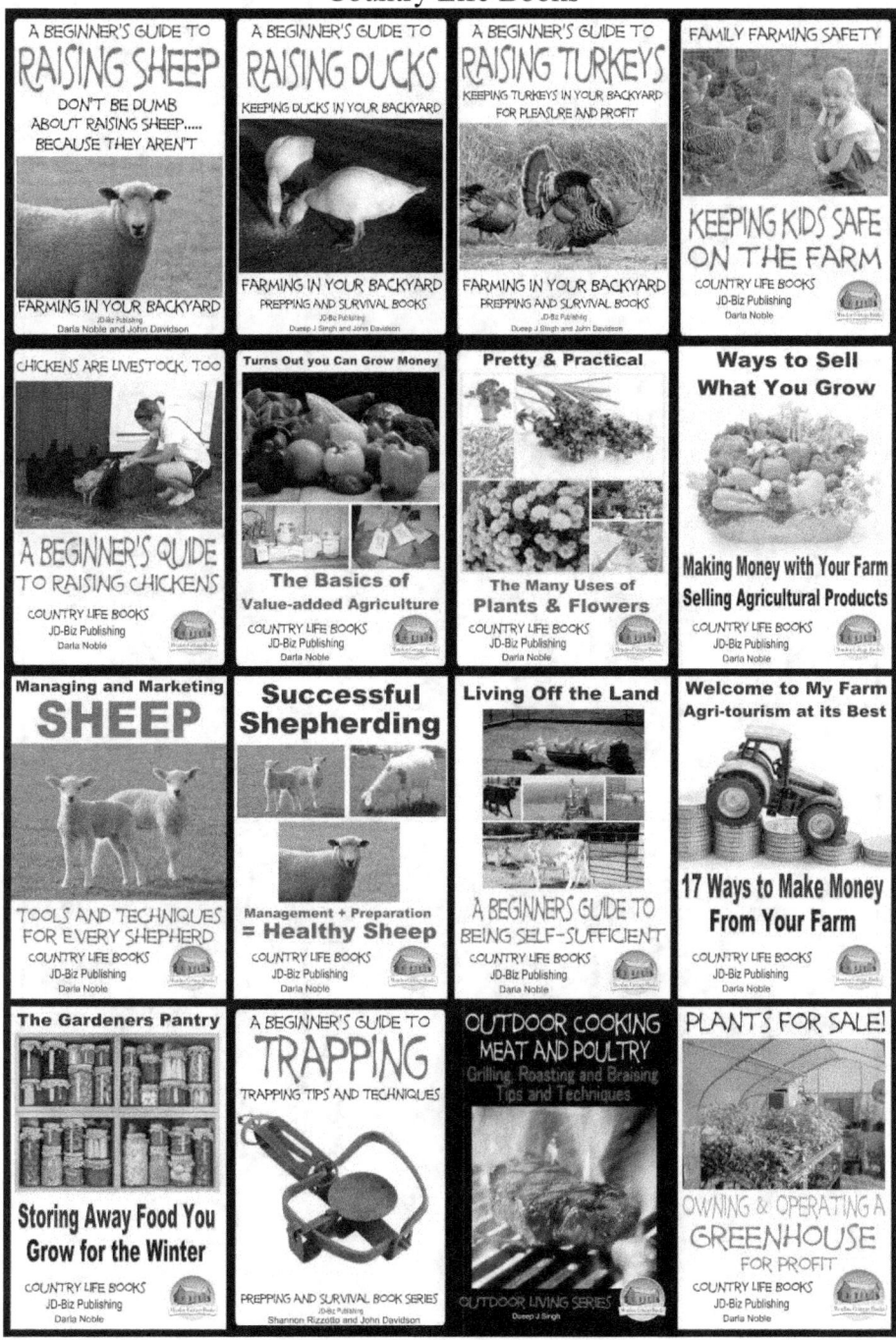

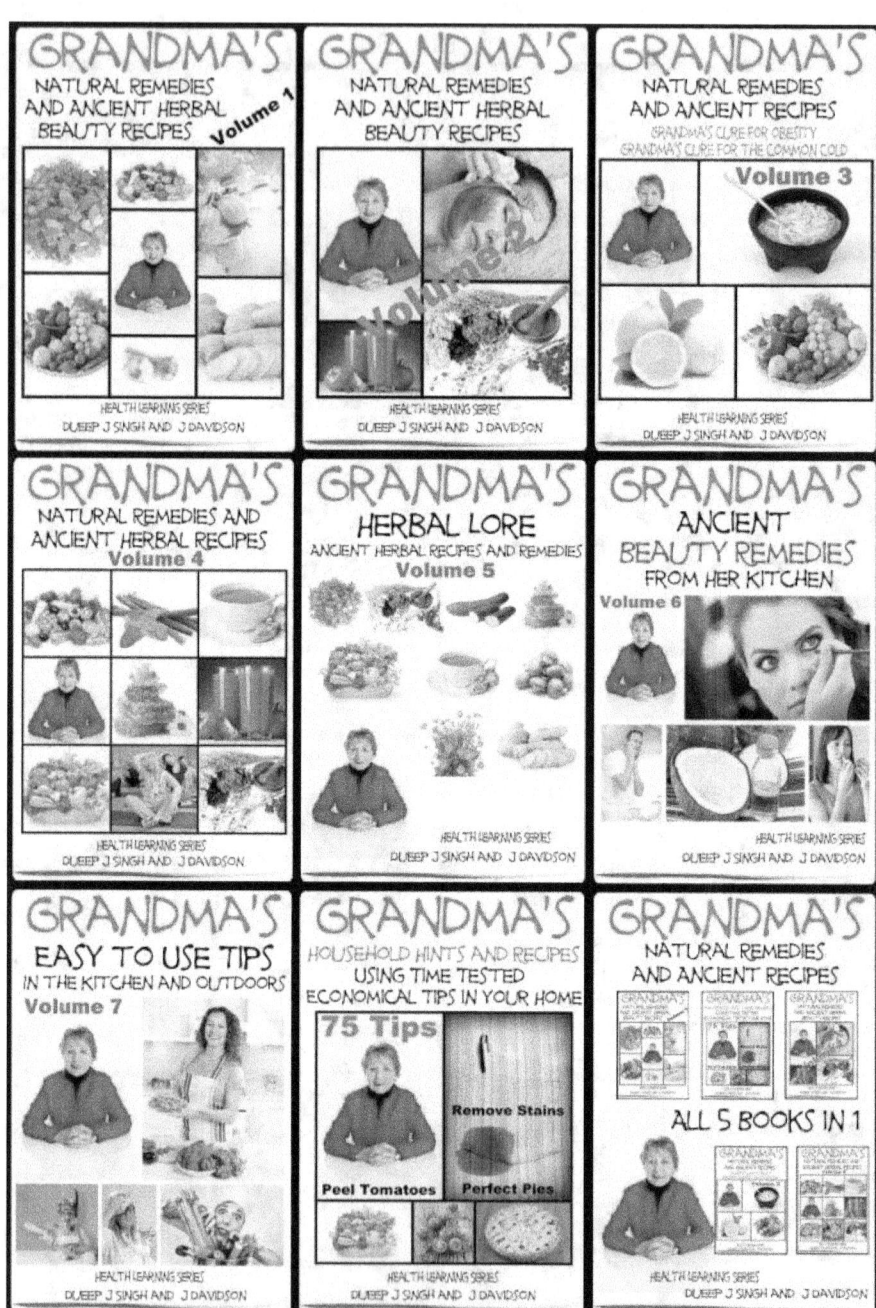

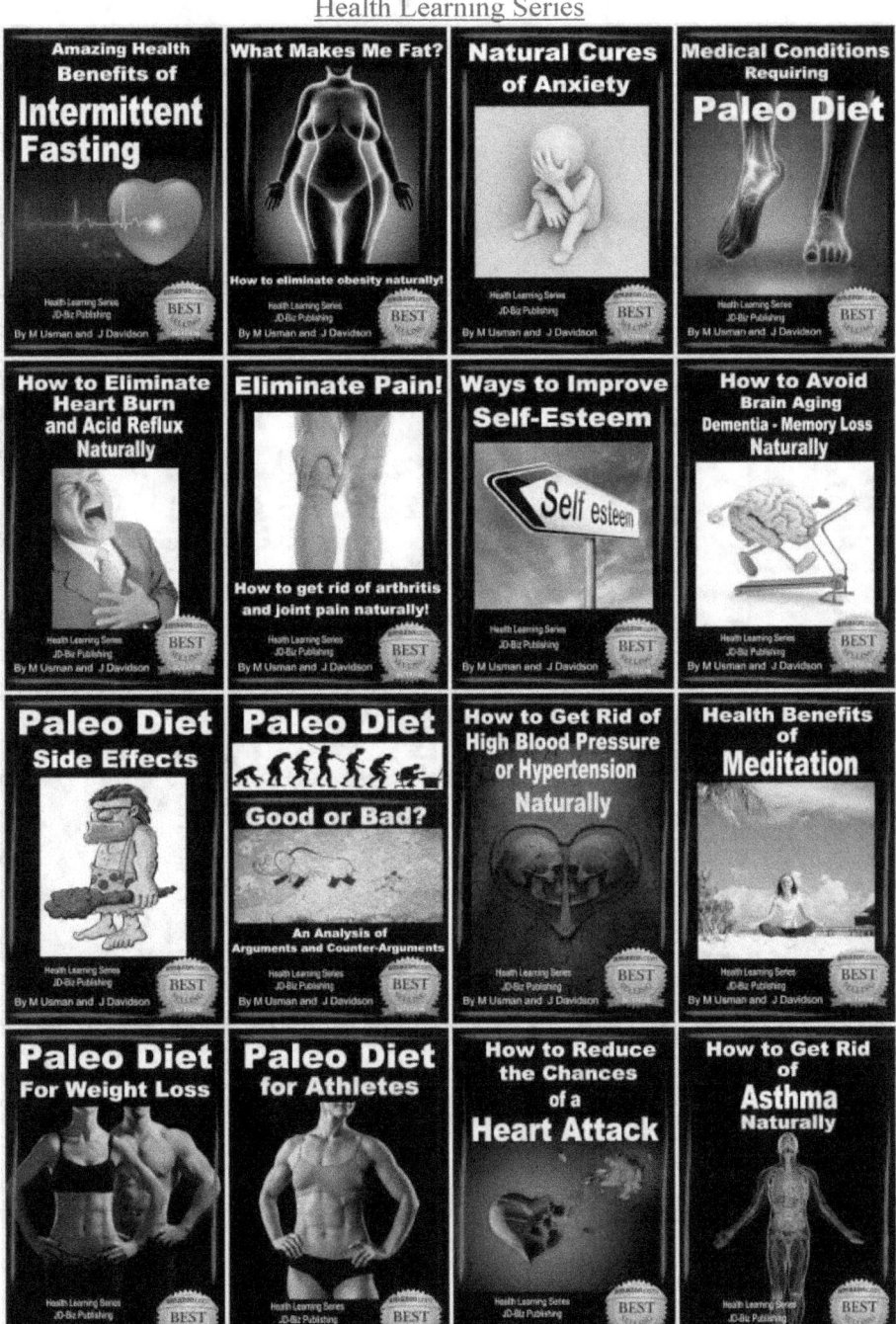

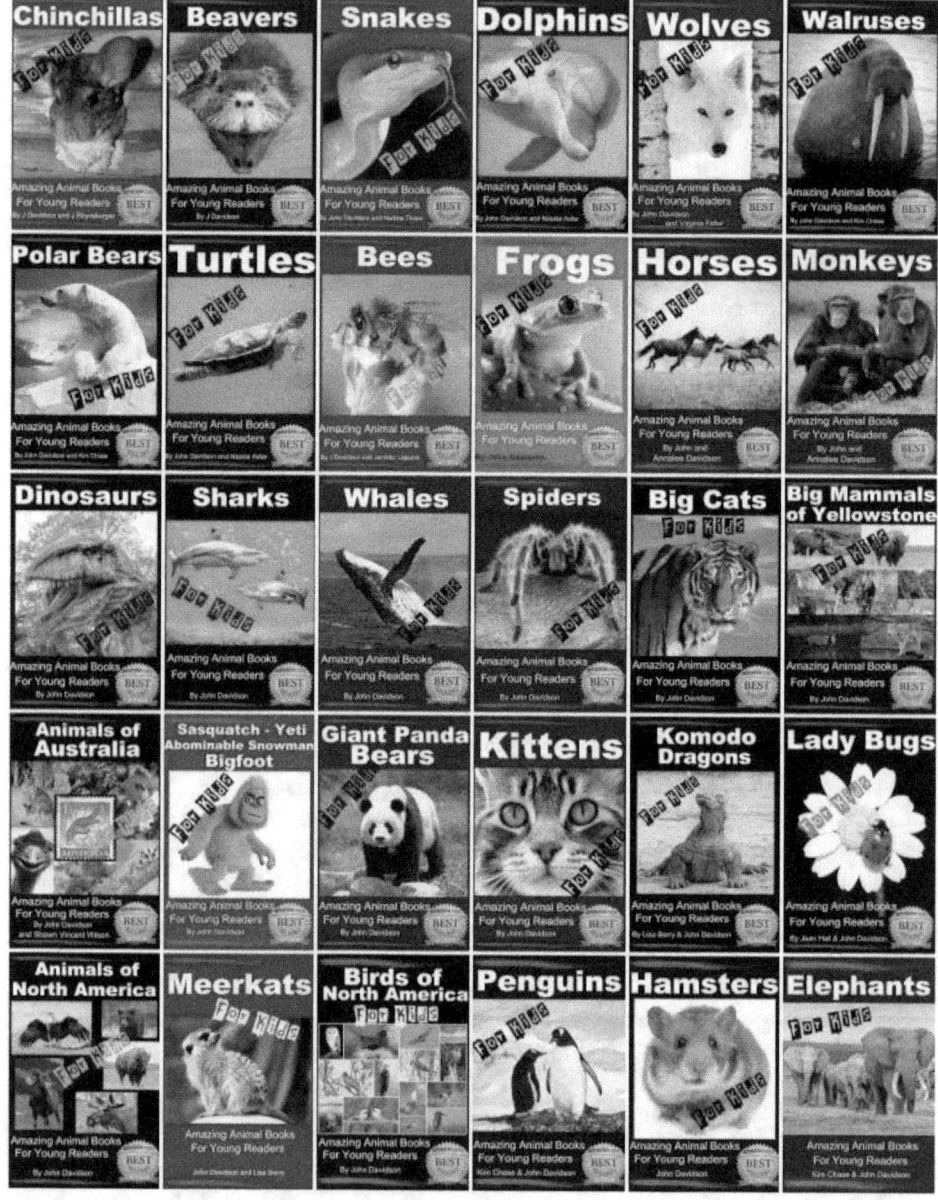

Learn To Draw Series

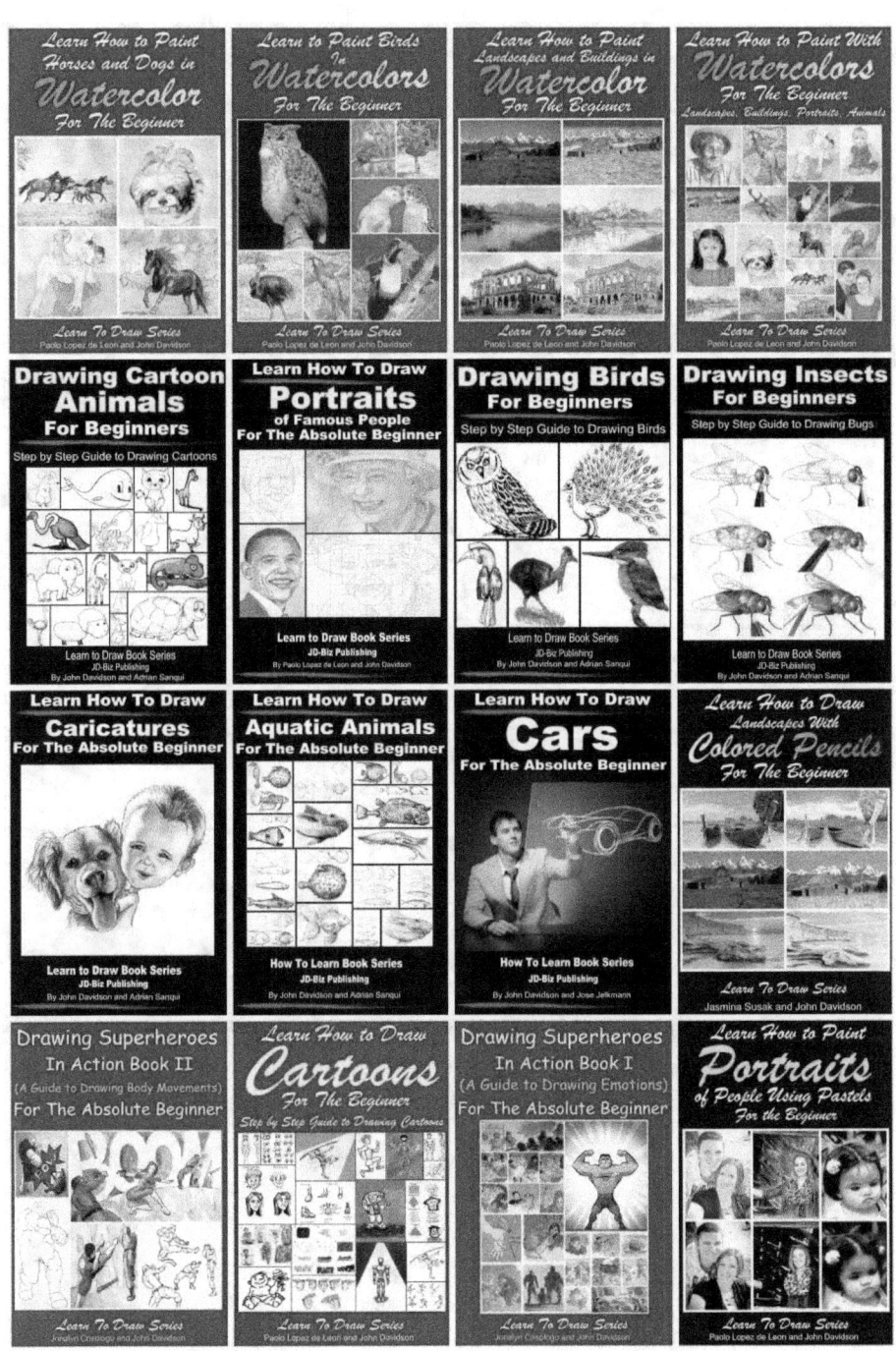

How to Build and Plan Books

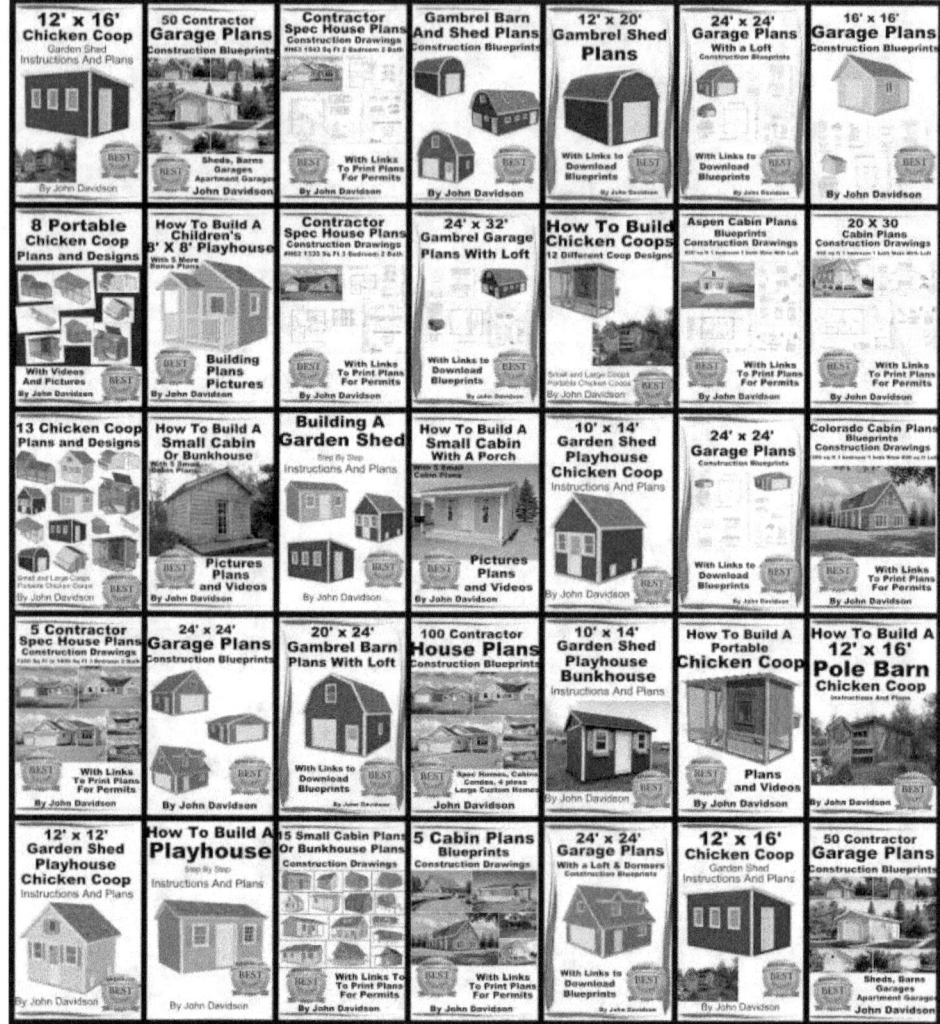

Entrepreneur Book Series

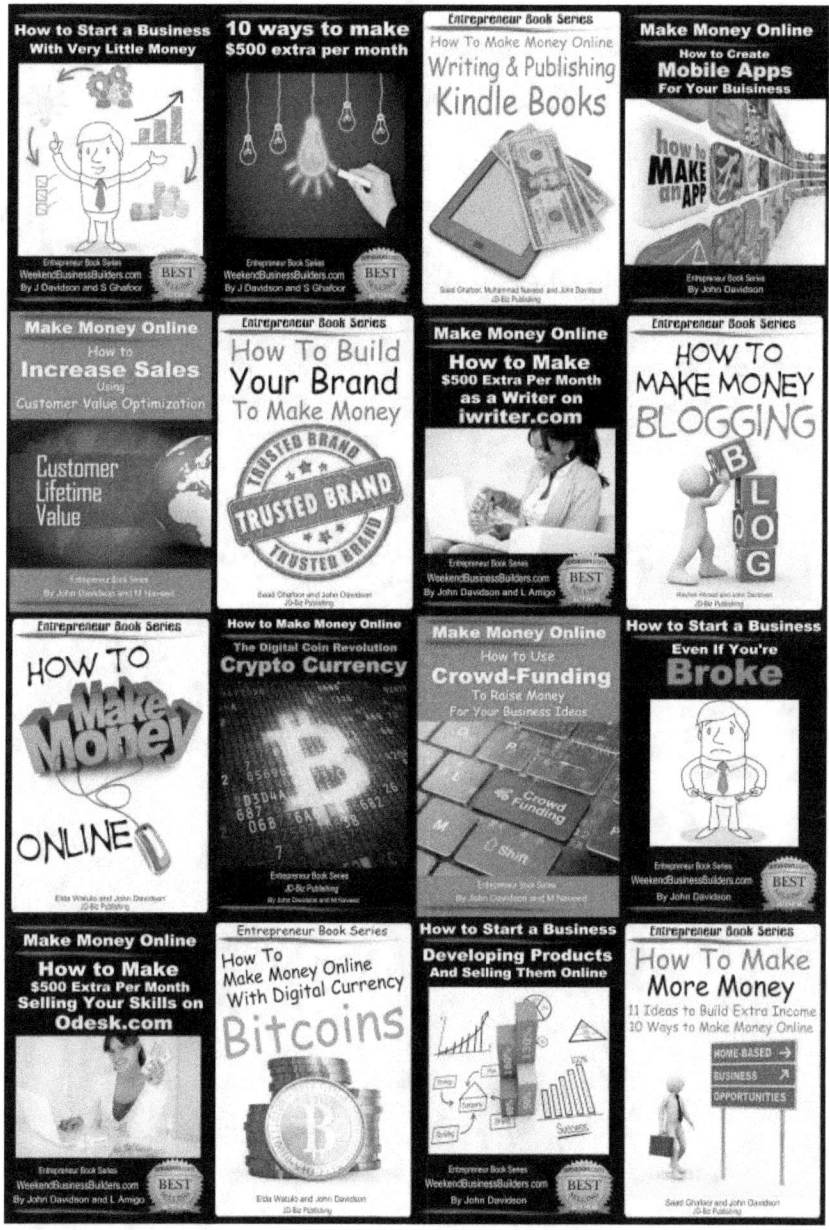

Our books are available at

1. Amazon.com

2. Barnes and Noble

3. Itunes

4. Kobo

5. Smashwords

6. Google Play Books

Download Free Books!

http://MendonCottageBooks.com

Publisher

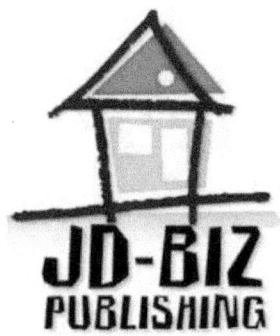

JD-Biz Corp

P O Box 374

Mendon, Utah 84325

http://www.jd-biz.com/

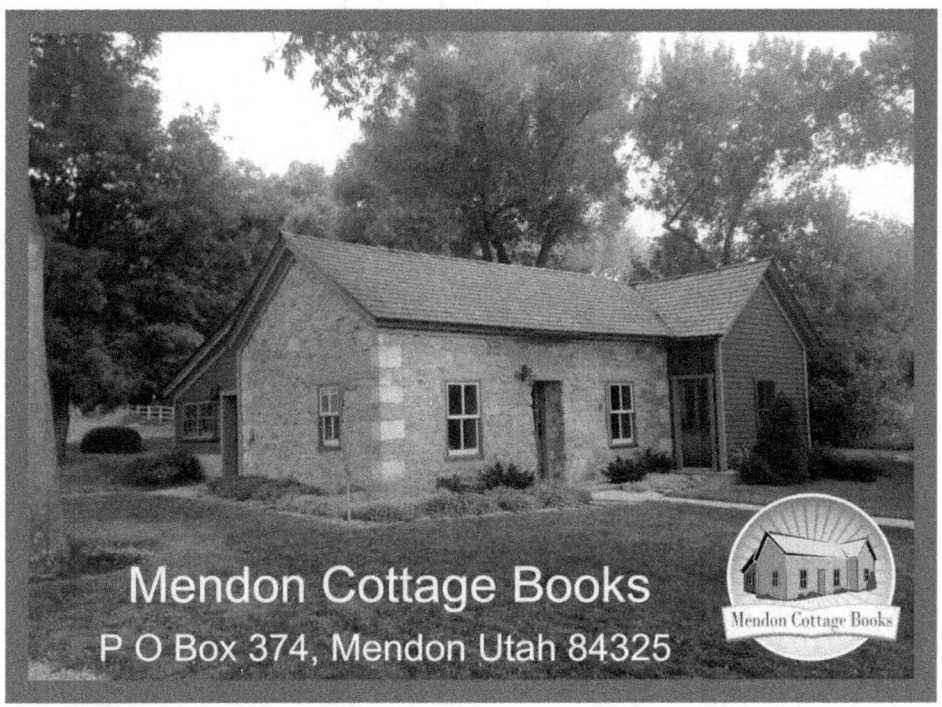

Mendon Cottage Books

P O Box 374, Mendon Utah 84325

www.ingramcontent.com/pod-product-compliance
Lightning Source LLC
Chambersburg PA
CBHW071146280526
45787CB00003B/1429